How To Become A Vertified Flight Instructor

Abraham Michael

Published by CEC Publisher, 2024.

This is a work of fiction. Similarities to real people, places, or events are entirely coincidental.

HOW TO BECOME A VERTIFIED FLIGHT INSTRUCTOR

First edition. March 7, 2024.

Copyright © 2024 Abraham Michael.

Written by Abraham Michael.

Table of Contents

How To Become A Vertified Flight Instructor

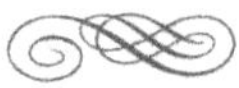

The Simple Guide to Learning Proper Technique
How To Become A Vertified Flight Instructor

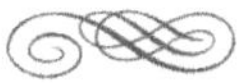

Abraham Michael

Disclaimer

While every precaution has been taken in the preparation of this book, the publisher assumes no responsibility for errors or omissions, or for damages resulting from the use of the information contained herein.

How To Become A Vertified Flight Instructor: The Simple Guide to Learning Proper Technique How To Become A Vertified Flight Instructor

First edition.

Disclaimer

I hope you find this exploration of post-flight debriefings insightful and comprehensive. If you have any specific points you'd like to add or modify, feel free to let me know.

Chapter 8

Foreword

IN THE DYNAMIC REALM of aviation, where precision and expertise soar to new heights, aspiring pilots seek the guidance of seasoned professionals to navigate the intricate path toward becoming a Certified Flight Instructor (CFI). In "How to Become a CFI," the author skillfully unveils the keys to mastery in this pivotal role, blending comprehensive knowledge with a passion for imparting it.

Drawing from years of firsthand experience, the author demystifies the complexities of flight instruction, offering a roadmap that goes beyond the regulatory requirements. This book is a compass for those on the journey to not only obtain a CFI certificate but to truly excel in the art and science of teaching aviation.

Readers will find within these pages a treasure trove of insights, from honing instructional techniques to fostering a deep understanding of aeronautical concepts. The author's commitment to cultivating effective educators in the cockpit is evident, creating a resource that transcends the status quo.

As aviation continually evolves, so too must its educators. This book serves as a beacon for those ready to embrace the challenges and rewards of guiding the next generation of aviators. Whether you're a seasoned pilot looking to transition to instructing or a fresh-faced enthusiast taking your first steps into the world of flight education, "How to Become a CFI" is an indispensable companion on your journey to excellence.

Prepare to embark on a transformative expedition, where knowledge meets passion, and teaching becomes an art form. This book is not just a guide; it's a testament to the profound impact a dedicated CFI can have on the aviation community. May your flight instructing endeavors be both enlightening and rewarding. Safe skies and happy teaching!

Abraham Michael

Abraham Michael

Introduction

Understanding the Role of a Certified Flight Instructor

The Significance of Flight Instruction in Aviation

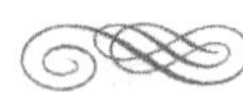

THE SIGNIFICANCE OF Flight Instruction in Aviation

Aviation stands as a testament to human innovation, connecting distant places and making the impossible a reality. At the heart of this extraordinary endeavor lies the pivotal role of flight instruction. It is not merely a process of transferring knowledge; it is the cornerstone upon which the entire aviation community builds its future.

A Foundation of Safety

In the dynamic world of aviation, safety is paramount. Flight instructors serve as the guardians of this principle, instilling a profound understanding of safety protocols from the very inception of a pilot's training. The significance of flight instruction is perhaps most evident in its ability to mold aviators with an unwavering commitment to safety, creating a culture that permeates every aspect of the industry.

Knowledge Transmission and Expertise Cultivation

Flight instruction is the conduit through which the wealth of aeronautical knowledge is transmitted to aspiring pilots. It goes beyond the mechanics of flight, encompassing meteorology, navigation, regulations, and a deep understanding of aircraft systems. The role of a flight instructor extends beyond the cockpit; it's a commitment to cultivating well-rounded aviators armed with comprehensive expertise.

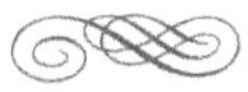

I'LL CONTINUE WITH the next part in the following response.

Responsibilities and Expectations of a CFI

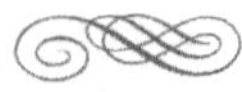

RESPONSIBILITIES AND Expectations of a CFI

Becoming a Certified Flight Instructor (CFI) is not just about mastering the technicalities of flight but embracing a role that goes beyond the cockpit. The responsibilities and expectations placed upon a CFI are multifaceted, shaping not only the future of individual aviators but influencing the broader landscape of aviation.

1. Safety Stewardship

At the core of a CFI's responsibilities lies a solemn commitment to safety. Beyond imparting the skills required for flight, a CFI must instill a deep-rooted sense of safety consciousness in their students. This extends from pre-flight checklists to emergency procedures, creating aviators who prioritize safety at every stage of their career.

2. Knowledge Transfer

The role of a CFI extends beyond being a skilled pilot; it transforms into that of an educator. A CFI must possess a comprehensive understanding of aeronautical concepts, regulations, and practical flying skills. The ability to transfer this knowledge effectively is paramount, ensuring that students not only pass exams but truly comprehend the intricacies of aviation.

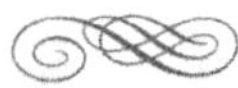

I'LL CONTINUE WITH the next part in the following response.

Chapter 1

Prerequisites and Preparation

Minimum Requirements for CFI Certification

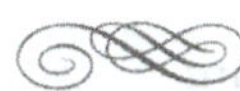

MINIMUM REQUIREMENTS for CFI Certification

Becoming a Certified Flight Instructor (CFI) is a significant milestone, symbolizing not only a mastery of aviation skills but a commitment to imparting that knowledge to future aviators. The journey to CFI certification involves meeting specific requirements that ensure a candidate is not only proficient in their flying abilities but also possesses the educational aptitude to guide others through the complexities of aviation.

1. Pilot Experience

The foundation for CFI certification is laid upon a solid base of pilot experience. The aspiring CFI must hold a commercial pilot certificate and demonstrate a depth of flight hours that exceeds the minimums required for lower-level certifications. This ensures that the candidate has encountered a variety of flying scenarios, building the necessary expertise to handle diverse situations that may arise during flight instruction.

2. Educational Background

While the aviation industry often emphasizes hands-on experience, a CFI candidate is expected to possess a strong educational foundation. A high school diploma or equivalent is a minimum requirement, ensuring that the candidate has the fundamental literacy and numeracy skills to convey complex aeronautical concepts in an understandable manner.

Building a Strong Foundation: Necessary Pilot Experience

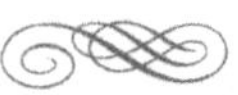

BUILDING A STRONG FOUNDATION: Necessary Pilot Experience

The journey to becoming a proficient Certified Flight Instructor (CFI) begins with a deliberate focus on building a robust foundation of pilot experience. This cornerstone is more than a mere prerequisite; it is the bedrock upon which the aspiring CFI constructs a wealth of knowledge and skills, preparing them to guide the next generation of aviators.

1. Accumulating Flight Hours

At the heart of pilot experience lies the accumulation of flight hours. Aspiring CFIs embark on a journey that goes beyond the minimums required for earlier certifications. The flight hours become not just a numerical benchmark but a narrative of diverse flying experiences — from navigating diverse weather conditions to mastering various aircraft types. Each hour logged represents a lesson learned, a challenge overcome, and a step closer to the pinnacle of flight instruction.

2. Diverse Flying Scenarios

A seasoned CFI is one who has been exposed to a multitude of flying scenarios. This entails more than routine flights under ideal conditions. It involves confronting adverse weather, managing complex airspace, and executing precise maneuvers under varying circumstances. This diversity cultivates adaptability, a trait essential for imparting practical insights to future aviators who will encounter a spectrum of challenges throughout their careers.

Selecting the Right Aircraft and Endorsements

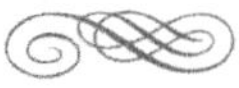

CERTAINLY, LET'S DELVE into the crucial topic of "Selecting the Right Aircraft and Endorsements."

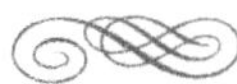

SELECTING THE RIGHT Aircraft and Endorsements

The choice of aircraft and the endorsements attached to a Certified Flight Instructor's (CFI) repertoire is a nuanced decision that shapes not only their teaching methodology but also the depth of knowledge they can impart to aspiring aviators. In this exploration, we dissect the considerations involved in selecting the right aircraft and endorsements, illuminating the path toward becoming a well-rounded CFI.

1. Understanding Student Needs

The foundation of selecting the right aircraft for instruction is rooted in understanding the needs of the students. Each aircraft type brings its own set of challenges and advantages. A knowledgeable CFI evaluates the training requirements of their students, considering factors such as mission profiles, future career paths, and individual learning preferences. This tailored approach ensures that the aircraft chosen aligns seamlessly with the student's journey into the skies.

2. Versatility in Aircraft Types

A seasoned CFI is adept at instructing across a spectrum of aircraft types. This versatility not only expands the CFI's own skill set but also enriches the training experience for their students. From nimble single-engine trainers to complex multi-engine aircraft, the ability to navigate and instruct in various platforms broadens the horizons of both the instructor and the aspiring pilot.

Chapter 2

Mastering Aeronautical Knowledg

Comprehensive Review of Aviation Regulations

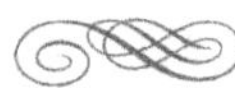

CERTAINLY, LET'S DELVE into the crucial topic of "Comprehensive Review of Aviation Regulations."

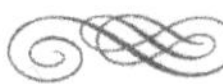

COMPREHENSIVE REVIEW of Aviation Regulations

In the intricate tapestry of aviation, regulations serve as the guiding threads that weave safety, order, and standardization into the fabric of the skies. For a Certified Flight Instructor (CFI), possessing a comprehensive understanding of aviation regulations is not merely a professional obligation; it is a commitment to nurturing a culture of safety, compliance, and excellence in the realm of flight instruction.

1. Foundations of Regulatory Knowledge

At the core of a CFI's responsibility is an intimate familiarity with the foundational regulatory documents that govern aviation. This includes, but is not limited to, the Federal Aviation Regulations (FARs) in the United States. A meticulous review and continuous update of these regulations are imperative to ensure that the instruction provided aligns seamlessly with the current legal framework.

2. Interpretation and Application

Regulations are not static; they are living documents that evolve with the dynamics of the aviation industry. A proficient CFI goes beyond rote memorization; they delve into the interpretation and application of regulations in real-world scenarios. This nuanced understanding allows them to impart not only what the regulations state but also why they exist and how they contribute to overall flight safety.

-Depth Understanding of Aerodynamics

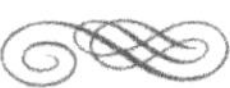

CERTAINLY, LET'S EXPLORE the intricate world of "Depth Understanding of Aerodynamics."

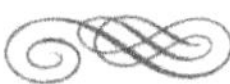

DEPTH UNDERSTANDING of Aerodynamics

In the celestial dance of flight, aerodynamics is the choreographer, orchestrating the harmonious balance between forces that propel an aircraft through the skies. For a Certified Flight Instructor (CFI), a profound understanding of aerodynamics is not a mere academic pursuit; it is the key to unlocking the mysteries of flight and, more importantly, the ability to convey these principles with clarity and precision.

1. Fundamentals of Lift and Drag

At the heart of aerodynamics lies the interplay of forces that govern an aircraft's ascent and descent. Lift, the force that defies gravity, and drag, the resistance that opposes forward motion, form the fundamental duo. A CFI must not only grasp these principles intimately but also possess the capability to distill these complex concepts into digestible knowledge for their students.

2. The Symphony of Airfoil Shape

Understanding aerodynamics transcends memorizing equations; it delves into the intricate nuances of airfoil shapes. From the elegant curve of a wing to the subtle manipulations that optimize lift, a CFI must navigate the intricacies of airfoil design. This knowledge becomes the lens through which they interpret the subtle dance between the aircraft and the air molecules it displaces.

3. Effects of Controls and Surfaces

A proficient CFI extends their expertise to the effects of controls and surfaces on an aircraft's behavior. How does altering the angle of attack influence lift? What role do ailerons, elevators, and rudders play in steering through the boundless expanse above? These questions form the basis of a CFI's instruction, shaping the practical understanding that transforms a pilot into a masterful aviator.

Navigating Weather Patterns and Meteorology

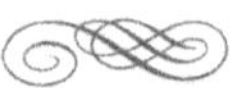

CERTAINLY, LET'S DELVE into the intricacies of "Navigating Weather Patterns and Meteorology."

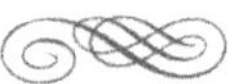

NAVIGATING WEATHER Patterns and Meteorology

In the ethereal expanse where earth and sky converge, understanding the language of clouds, winds, and atmospheric phenomena is an indispensable skill for any aviator, particularly a Certified Flight Instructor (CFI). Navigating weather patterns and mastering meteorology is not just about predicting storms; it is about instilling in pilots a profound awareness of the ever-changing canvas that is the sky.

1. Decoding the Atmosphere

Meteorology begins with decoding the language of the atmosphere, a complex ballet of air masses, pressure systems, and temperature differentials. For a CFI, this is more than a theoretical exercise; it's the ability to translate these atmospheric nuances into actionable insights for pilots. From high-pressure systems to the subtleties of temperature inversions, a CFI becomes a meteorological translator, helping pilots make informed decisions in the sky.

2. Understanding Weather Hazards

The skies, while enchanting, can harbor hazards that demand a vigilant eye. Thunderstorms, turbulence, icing – a CFI must be well-versed in identifying and mitigating these potential dangers. The art of meteorology is not just about predicting weather; it's about imparting a proactive mindset, teaching pilots to read the signs nature provides and respond with calculated precision.

3. Practical Weather Decision-Making

Weather patterns are not static; they are dynamic, evolving entities that demand continuous evaluation. A seasoned CFI doesn't just teach meteorology as a series of facts but as a skill set for making real-time decisions. Whether it's altering a flight plan based on developing weather conditions or deciding when it's safest to postpone a lesson, a CFI's expertise extends beyond the classroom, preparing pilots for the ever-shifting tapestry of the sky.

Chapter 3

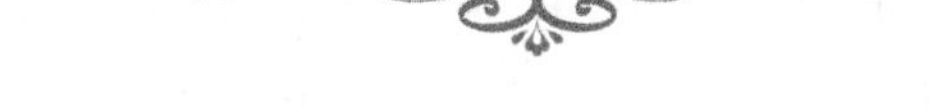

Effective Teaching Techniques

Pedagogical Strategies for Flight Instructors

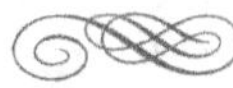

CERTAINLY, LET'S EXPLORE the art of "Pedagogical Strategies for Flight Instructors."

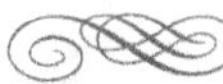

PEDAGOGICAL STRATEGIES for Flight Instructors

In the realm of flight instruction, mastery extends beyond the cockpit; it encompasses the art of effective teaching. A Certified Flight Instructor (CFI) is not only a skilled aviator but also a mentor, guiding aspiring pilots through the complexities of aviation. The pedagogical strategies employed by CFIs are the keystones that unlock understanding, shape proficiency, and cultivate a passion for flight.

1. Individualized Instruction

The diversity among aspiring pilots is vast, encompassing varied learning styles, backgrounds, and aptitudes. A seasoned CFI recognizes this heterogeneity and tailors their instruction to individual needs. Whether it's adapting explanations to resonate with visual learners or providing hands-on experiences for those who thrive through practice, individualized instruction is the cornerstone of effective teaching.

2. Creating a Collaborative Environment

Learning to fly is not a solitary endeavor; it's a collaborative journey between instructor and student. A skilled CFI fosters an environment where questions are encouraged, curiosity is nurtured, and mistakes are viewed as opportunities for growth. This collaborative approach transforms the learning process from a series of tasks to a shared exploration of the skies.

3. Practical Application of Theoretical Concepts

Aviation is a fusion of theory and practice, and effective CFIs bridge this gap seamlessly. Rather than presenting theoretical concepts in isolation, they weave practical applications into every lesson. Whether explaining the principles of navigation during a cross-country flight or illustrating aerodynamics during maneuvers, CFIs ensure that theoretical knowledge is not an abstract concept but a tangible tool for aviators.

4. Harnessing Technological Resources

In the modern era, technology is a potent ally in the realm of flight instruction. CFIs adeptly integrate flight simulators, digital resources, and interactive tools to enhance the learning experience. These technological aids provide a dynamic platform for students to practice, receive feedback, and develop the muscle memory crucial for safe and precise flying.

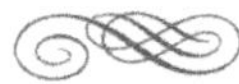

I'LL CONTINUE WITH the next part in the following response.

Tailoring Instruction to Individual Learning Styles

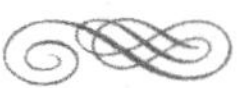

CERTAINLY, LET'S DELVE into the intricate art of "Tailoring Instruction to Individual Learning Styles."

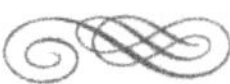

TAILORING INSTRUCTION to Individual Learning Styles

In the realm of flight instruction, recognizing the uniqueness of each aspiring pilot is not just a pedagogical choice; it's an imperative for success. The ability to tailor instruction to individual learning styles is a hallmark of an exceptional Certified Flight Instructor (CFI), transcending the conventional model of one-size-fits-all education and paving the way for a personalized journey into the skies.

1. Understanding Learning Preferences

Every student who embarks on the journey to become a pilot brings a distinct set of learning preferences to the cockpit. Some thrive on visual stimuli, absorbing information through charts and diagrams, while others grasp concepts more readily through hands-on experiences. A discerning CFI actively engages with their students, discerning their learning preferences through observation, communication, and mutual exploration.

2. Visual Learners: Charting the Skies

For visual learners, the sky is a canvas, and charts and diagrams are the brushstrokes that paint a vivid understanding of flight. CFIs adept at tailoring instruction to visual learners leverage tools such as sectional charts, navigation diagrams, and visual aids to elucidate complex concepts. Whether it's plotting a course or understanding airspace, visual learners find their pathway through the skies illuminated by the strategic use of graphical representation.

3. Auditory Learners: The Symphony of Aviation

The hum of an aircraft's engine, the rhythmic dance of control surfaces – for auditory learners, aviation is a symphony waiting to be heard. CFIs attuned to this learning style incorporate oral explanations, verbal discussions, and interactive dialogues into their lessons. By verbalizing concepts, explaining procedures, and fostering open communication, auditory learners find resonance in the language of flight.

4. Kinesthetic Learners: Embracing Hands-On Experience

Kinesthetic learners crave the tactile experience of manipulating controls, feeling the forces of flight firsthand. CFIs catering to this learning style integrate hands-on experiences into their lessons, utilizing flight simulators, conducting interactive exercises, and emphasizing practical application. The cockpit becomes a classroom where kinesthetic learners can translate theoretical knowledge into physical mastery.

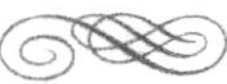

I'LL CONTINUE WITH the next part in the following response.

Creating Engaging Lesson Plans

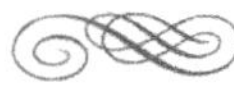

CERTAINLY, LET'S EXPLORE the art of "Creating Engaging Lesson Plans."

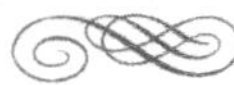

CREATING ENGAGING LESSON Plans

The essence of flight instruction lies not just in imparting knowledge but in crafting an experience that resonates with aspiring aviators. Certified Flight Instructors (CFIs) wield a unique responsibility in shaping lesson plans that go beyond the ordinary, fostering engagement, curiosity, and a passion for flight. The art of creating engaging lesson plans is the canvas upon which the journey into the skies is painted.

1. Setting Clear Objectives

A well-structured lesson plan begins with clearly defined objectives. What skills should the student acquire? What knowledge is essential for their progression? CFIs meticulously outline these objectives, providing a roadmap that guides both instructor and student through the intricacies of the lesson. Clear objectives not only streamline the learning process but also serve as motivational milestones for the aspiring pilot.

2. Incorporating Real-World Scenarios

Flight instruction is not a detached exercise in theory; it is a preparation for real-world scenarios. Engaging lesson plans immerse students in practical applications, simulating scenarios they may encounter in actual flight. Whether it's navigating through changing weather conditions or handling emergency procedures, students are not just learning concepts but developing the critical thinking skills required for safe aviation.

3. Utilizing Interactive Technologies

The modern era brings a plethora of interactive technologies that can elevate the learning experience. Flight simulators, virtual reality, and digital resources offer immersive opportunities for students to apply theoretical knowledge in a dynamic environment. CFIs adept at incorporating these technologies into their lesson plans create an interactive, hands-on experience that resonates with the tech-savvy generation of aspiring pilots.

4. Promoting Student Involvement

Engagement thrives in an environment where students actively participate in their own learning. CFIs design lesson plans that encourage questions, discussions, and collaborative problem-solving. This active involvement transforms the learning process from a passive reception of information to a shared exploration, where both instructor and student contribute to the unfolding narrative of each lesson.

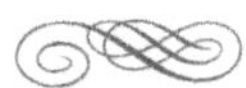

Chapter 4

Practical Flight Instruction

Developing Proficiency in Maneuvers and Procedures

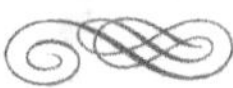

CERTAINLY, LET'S EXPLORE the journey of "Developing Proficiency in Maneuvers and Procedures."

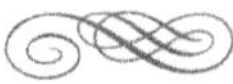

DEVELOPING PROFICIENCY in Maneuvers and Procedures

Becoming a skilled aviator transcends the mastery of flight controls; it entails a seamless integration of maneuvers and procedures that define the artistry of flying. Certified Flight Instructors (CFIs) play a pivotal role in sculpting this proficiency, guiding aspiring pilots through a meticulously crafted curriculum that transforms theoretical knowledge into practical expertise.

1. Foundations of Basic Maneuvers

Proficiency begins with a solid foundation in basic maneuvers. CFIs delve into the intricacies of climbs, descents, turns, and stalls, emphasizing not just the mechanical execution but the underlying principles that govern these actions. This foundational knowledge forms the bedrock upon which more advanced maneuvers and procedures are built.

2. Precision in Takeoffs and Landings

Takeoffs and landings are the alpha and omega of flight, demanding a level of precision that goes beyond routine procedures. CFIs instill in their students the art of gauging distances, adjusting for wind, and executing flawless takeoffs and landings. These seemingly routine maneuvers are, in essence, a canvas for developing the muscle memory and instinctual judgment essential for safe and competent piloting.

3. Navigating the Three-Dimensional Space

Flight is a dance through the three-dimensional canvas of the sky, requiring pilots to master maneuvers that transcend the limitations of two-dimensional thinking. From steep turns that challenge the boundaries of coordination to spiraling descents that demand a nuanced understanding of energy management, CFIs guide their students through the symphony of controlled flight.

4. Emergency Procedures and Simulations

Proficiency is not complete without the ability to respond decisively in the face of unexpected challenges. CFIs introduce emergency procedures, from engine failures to instrument malfunctions, in a simulated yet realistic environment. These simulations not only prepare students for real-world contingencies but also cultivate the mental resilience required for confident decision-making under pressure.

5. Cross-Country Navigation

Navigating the vast expanse between departure and destination is a rite of passage for every aviator. CFIs structure lessons that go beyond point-to-point navigation, incorporating the nuances of cross-country flight. This includes flight planning, navigation techniques, and the ability to adapt to changing weather conditions – skills that transform pilots into adept navigators of the skies.

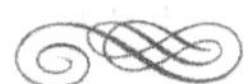

Conducting Safe and Structured Flight Lessons

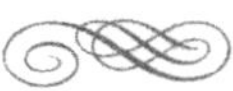

CERTAINLY, LET'S EXPLORE the imperative aspects of "Conducting Safe and Structured Flight Lessons."

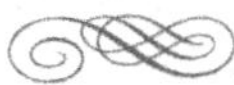

CONDUCTING SAFE AND Structured Flight Lessons

In the delicate dance between the earth and the sky, the role of a Certified Flight Instructor (CFI) extends beyond imparting knowledge; it encompasses the responsibility of conducting flight lessons that are not only educational but also safe, structured, and transformative. The canvas of the sky is the classroom, and the lessons taught within its expanse echo the ethos of professionalism, precision, and a commitment to shaping competent aviators.

1. Pre-flight Briefings: The Foundation of Safety

Every safe flight begins on the ground, and CFIs understand the significance of thorough pre-flight briefings. These sessions are not mere rituals but a meticulous examination of weather conditions, aircraft status, and flight plans. CFIs instill in their students the habit of comprehensive pre-flight assessments, cultivating a mindset where safety is not negotiable.

2. Structured Lesson Plans: Navigating the Skies Methodically

Structure is the backbone of effective flight lessons. CFIs meticulously craft lesson plans that follow a logical progression, building upon previously acquired skills. This structured approach ensures that students are not overwhelmed but instead experience a gradual and systematic immersion into the complexities of aviation. Each lesson is a building block, laying the foundation for the next stage of proficiency.

3. In-Flight Communication: The Art of Instruction

Communication in the cockpit is not just about conveying information; it's an art form that demands clarity, precision, and adaptability. CFIs are adept at articulating instructions concisely, providing real-time feedback, and fostering an open channel of communication. This artistry in instruction transforms the cockpit into a dynamic learning environment where every word carries significance.

4. Emergency Preparedness: Navigating Unforeseen Challenges

A key facet of safe flight lessons is preparing students for the unexpected. CFIs incorporate emergency procedures into their curriculum, simulating scenarios that demand quick thinking and decisive action. This proactive approach not only hones students' ability to handle emergencies but also instills in them the confidence that comes from thorough preparation.

5. Post-flight Debriefings: Reflection and Improvement

The learning process extends beyond the touchdown; it continues in the reflective moments of post-flight debriefings. CFIs engage in comprehensive discussions with their students, analyzing the flight from takeoff to landing. These debriefings are not critiques but collaborative reflections, identifying strengths, addressing challenges, and fostering a continuous cycle of improvement.

Utilizing Simulators for Enhanced Training

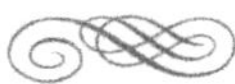

CERTAINLY, LET'S EXPLORE the transformative realm of "Utilizing Simulators for Enhanced Training."

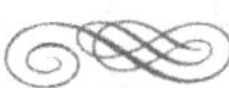

UTILIZING SIMULATORS for Enhanced Training

In the ever-evolving landscape of aviation education, the integration of cutting-edge technology has become not just a luxury but a necessity. Among the myriad tools at the disposal of Certified Flight Instructors (CFIs), simulators stand out as powerful allies in sculpting skilled aviators. This exploration delves into the multifaceted advantages, nuances, and strategic applications of utilizing simulators for enhanced flight training.

1. Realism in a Virtual Realm

Simulators are no longer mere imitations; they are portals to realistic virtual realms. The advancements in simulation technology have reached a point where the line between the virtual and the tangible blurs. From cockpit layouts to instrument panels, simulators replicate the nuances of real aircraft, providing an immersive experience that transcends the limitations of traditional ground-based training.

2. Risk Mitigation: Learning from Mistakes Safely

Aviation, by its nature, leaves little room for errors. Simulators, however, offer a unique sanctuary where mistakes are not only permissible but encouraged. CFIs leverage simulated environments to expose students to a spectrum of challenging scenarios – engine failures, adverse weather conditions, and emergency procedures. It's a controlled space where errors become invaluable lessons without real-world consequences.

3. Procedural Proficiency: From Theory to Muscle Memory

The transition from theoretical knowledge to procedural proficiency is a pivotal phase in flight training. Simulators provide a dynamic platform for students to translate theoretical concepts into muscle memory. From pre-flight checklists to intricate maneuvers, the repetitive practice within a simulator fosters the precision and instinctual response required for safe and confident piloting.

4. Scenario-Based Training: Navigating Complexity

The unpredictable nature of aviation demands a training approach that mirrors this complexity. Simulators allow CFIs to craft scenario-based training, presenting students with dynamic challenges that go beyond the confines of routine exercises. Navigating through changing weather conditions, responding to air traffic control instructions, and managing system failures become integral components of simulator-based scenarios.

5. Instrument Proficiency: Mastering Avionics

As aviation technology advances, so does the complexity of onboard avionics. Simulators serve as laboratories where students can master the intricacies of modern instrument panels. Whether it's practicing instrument approaches, interpreting navigation displays, or managing autopilot systems, simulators provide a risk-free environment for honing instrument proficiency.

6. Time and Cost Efficiency: Maximizing Resources

Flight time is a precious commodity in aviation education, and simulators offer a strategic solution to maximize its efficacy. While actual flight hours remain indispensable, simulators allow for focused skill development without the constraints of fuel costs and aircraft availability. CFIs optimize training schedules, ensuring that every minute spent in the cockpit is purposeful and targeted.

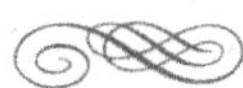

I'LL CONTINUE WITH the next part in the following response.

Chapter 5

Communication and Feedback

Building Rapport with Students

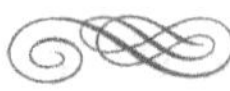

CERTAINLY, LET'S EXPLORE the delicate art of "Building Rapport with Students."

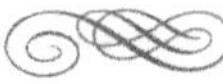

BUILDING RAPPORT WITH Students

In the realm of flight instruction, where the sky is both classroom and canvas, the relationship between a Certified Flight Instructor (CFI) and their students transcends the boundaries of traditional education. Beyond the technicalities of avionics and maneuvers, the success of flight training hinges on a less tangible yet equally crucial element – the rapport between instructor and student. This exploration delves into the nuances of building meaningful connections that foster trust, communication, and a shared passion for the skies.

1. Establishing an Open Line of Communication

Communication is the cornerstone of any successful instructional relationship. CFIs initiate the journey of rapport by creating an environment where communication is not a one-way street but a dynamic exchange. From the very first pre-flight briefing, students are encouraged to voice their questions, concerns, and aspirations, setting the stage for a collaborative and open learning experience.

2. Understanding Individual Learning Styles

Each student is a unique entity with distinct learning preferences and styles. CFIs invest time in understanding these individual nuances, tailoring their instructional approach to match the cognitive and practical preferences of each student. Whether it's visual aids, hands-on experiences, or verbal explanations, adapting to diverse learning styles ensures that the lessons resonate effectively.

3. Fostering a Positive Learning Environment

The cockpit is not just a mechanical space; it's a learning environment that should radiate positivity and encouragement. CFIs infuse their lessons with a sense of enthusiasm, cultivating an atmosphere where mistakes are viewed as stepping stones to improvement, and accomplishments are celebrated. This positive reinforcement extends beyond the aircraft, creating a ripple effect that influences the broader mindset of the aspiring aviator.

4. Personalizing the Learning Journey

Flight training is not a one-size-fits-all endeavor. CFIs weave a personalized narrative into the learning journey, relating concepts to the individual goals and aspirations of each student. Whether it's a dream of becoming a commercial pilot, a passion for aerobatics, or an ambition to fly recreationally, CFIs align their guidance with the unique trajectory of each student, making the learning experience both relevant and personally meaningful.

5. Navigating Challenges with Empathy

The path to becoming a pilot is punctuated with challenges – from mastering complex maneuvers to overcoming moments of self-doubt. CFIs approach these challenges not just as technical hurdles but as human experiences. Empathy becomes a guiding force, allowing instructors to navigate the emotional highs and lows of the learning curve with sensitivity and understanding.

6. Encouraging Continuous Feedback

Rapport flourishes in an environment where feedback is not just welcomed but actively encouraged. CFIs establish a culture of continuous improvement, inviting students to share their perspectives on lessons, communication styles, and overall experiences. This feedback loop becomes a catalyst for refining instructional approaches, ensuring that the learning journey remains a collaborative evolution.

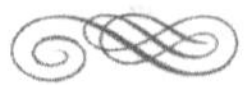

Providing Constructive Feedback

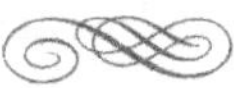

CERTAINLY, LET'S EXPLORE the art and importance of "Providing Constructive Feedback."

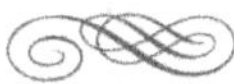

PROVIDING CONSTRUCTIVE Feedback

In the intricate dance of flight instruction, where the quest for mastery is as vast as the skies, the role of constructive feedback emerges as a linchpin. Certified Flight Instructors (CFIs) navigate the delicate balance of nurturing growth while addressing areas for improvement. This exploration delves into the nuances of providing feedback that transcends critique, fostering an environment of continuous learning and mastery in the journey to becoming a skilled aviator.

1. The Purposeful Lens of Improvement

Constructive feedback is not a mere assessment; it's a lens through which both instructor and student view the path to improvement. CFIs approach feedback sessions with a purposeful mindset, recognizing that each nugget of critique is an opportunity for refinement. The emphasis is not on shortcomings alone but on the constructive steps that lead to enhanced proficiency.

2. Timely and Specific: A Precision Approach

Feedback loses its efficacy when it is vague or delayed. CFIs prioritize the timeliness and specificity of their feedback, ensuring that it aligns with recent experiences in the cockpit. Specificity is the keystone – whether pinpointing a particular maneuver, communication skill, or decision-making process, the precision of feedback is what transforms it from an observation into a catalyst for improvement.

3. Balancing Positivity and Improvement Areas

The art of providing constructive feedback lies in striking a delicate balance between acknowledging achievements and addressing areas for improvement. CFIs adopt a positive framing, ensuring that commendations for successful maneuvers and adherence to procedures are woven seamlessly with insights on how to elevate performance further. This balance sustains motivation while fostering a commitment to excellence.

4. Tailoring Feedback to Individual Learning Styles

Just as instruction is tailored to individual learning styles, so too is feedback. CFIs recognize that each student processes and responds to feedback differently. Whether it's a preference for visual aids, hands-on demonstrations, or verbal discussions, tailoring the delivery of feedback to align with individual learning styles enhances its impact and resonance.

5. Encouraging Self-Reflection

Constructive feedback is a collaborative endeavor, inviting students to actively engage in the process of self-reflection. CFIs guide students to assess their own performances, encouraging them to identify areas where improvement is sought. This self-reflective component transforms feedback into a dialogue, fostering a sense of ownership over one's progress.

6. Setting Achievable Goals

Feedback is not just a reflection on past performance; it's a roadmap for future achievements. CFIs collaborate with students to set achievable and measurable goals based on the feedback received. These goals become beacons, guiding the trajectory of the learning journey and providing tangible milestones for continuous improvement.

7. Creating a Growth Mindset

Constructive feedback is not a static judgment but a dynamic catalyst for growth. CFIs instill in their students a growth mindset, emphasizing that every challenge, every critique, is an opportunity to evolve. This mindset shift transforms feedback from a potential source of anxiety into a source of motivation and resilience.

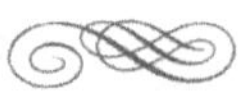

Addressing Common Student Challenges

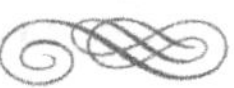

CERTAINLY, LET'S EXPLORE the nuanced task of "Addressing Common Student Challenges."

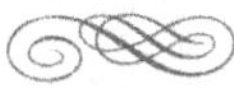

ADDRESSING COMMON STUDENT Challenges

In the intricate tapestry of flight training, students embark on a journey that unfolds amidst the hum of aircraft engines and the boundless expanse of the sky. Yet, this path to piloting prowess is not without its challenges. Certified Flight Instructors (CFIs) don the hat of mentors and guides, addressing common hurdles that aspiring aviators may encounter. This exploration navigates through these challenges, offering insights and strategies to empower both students and instructors in their pursuit of aviation excellence.

1. Overcoming Anxiety and Nervousness

The cockpit, with its array of controls and the weight of responsibility, can be an intimidating space for new aviators. CFIs recognize the prevalence of anxiety and nervousness among students and employ a multifaceted approach. From fostering a positive learning environment to gradual exposure to flying scenarios, strategies are woven into the fabric of instruction to ease students into the rhythm of flight.

2. Mastering Communication in the Sky

Effective communication between pilot and instructor is paramount in the cockpit. However, the airborne environment introduces unique challenges to verbal exchanges. CFIs address this challenge by integrating focused communication drills into training sessions. From concise radio communications to non-verbal cues, students are equipped with the tools to articulate their intentions and comprehend instructions with clarity.

3. Navigating Weather-Related Concerns

The unpredictability of weather is a formidable adversary in aviation. CFIs recognize that understanding and navigating weather patterns can be a daunting task for students. Weather-related challenges are met with comprehensive lessons on meteorology, enabling students to decipher forecasts, interpret weather charts, and make informed decisions regarding flight safety.

4. Developing Proficiency in Maneuvers and Procedures

Mastery of maneuvers and adherence to procedural protocols are pivotal aspects of pilot proficiency. CFIs, attuned to the learning curve, structure lessons that break down complex maneuvers into digestible components. Simulators become invaluable tools for students to refine their skills in a controlled environment before taking to the skies, fostering confidence and competence.

5. Balancing Theory and Practical Application

Theoretical knowledge is the bedrock upon which practical flying skills are built. Yet, finding the equilibrium between theory and application can be a challenge. CFIs bridge this gap by intertwining theoretical lessons with practical scenarios. Ground school sessions are not mere lectures but interactive discussions that connect theoretical concepts to real-world aviation scenarios, enriching the learning experience.

6. Cultivating Decision-Making Skills

Aviation demands split-second decision-making skills that weigh heavily on flight safety. CFIs guide students in the cultivation of this critical aptitude by incorporating scenario-based training. From simulated emergencies to navigating complex airspace, students are immersed in scenarios that demand quick thinking and precise decision-making, nurturing their ability to respond effectively under pressure.

7. Managing Time and Workload Effectively

The cockpit is a dynamic space where time is often of the essence. CFIs recognize the importance of instilling effective time management skills in their students. From pre-flight preparations to in-flight multitasking, students are coached to streamline their workflows, ensuring that they can navigate the demands of piloting with efficiency.

8. Building Resilience in the Face of Setbacks

Setbacks are an inevitable part of the learning journey. Whether it's a challenging maneuver or an unexpected change in weather conditions, students may face moments of frustration. CFIs act as mentors, fostering resilience by reframing setbacks as opportunities for growth. Debriefing sessions become constructive dialogues that extract lessons from challenges, transforming setbacks into stepping stones toward mastery.

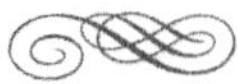

I'LL CONTINUE WITH the next part in the following response.

Chapter 6

The Art of Briefings and Debriefings

Pre-Flight Briefings: Setting the Stage for Success

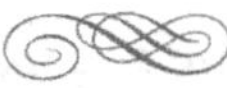

CERTAINLY, LET'S DELVE into the critical practice of "Pre-Flight Briefings: Setting the Stage for Success."

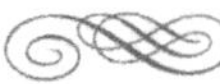

PRE-FLIGHT BRIEFINGS: Setting the Stage for Success

In the realm of aviation, where precision is paramount and safety is non-negotiable, the pre-flight briefing stands as a cornerstone of every successful journey into the skies. Certified Flight Instructors (CFIs) understand that the minutes spent on the ground before takeoff are instrumental in shaping the outcome of the entire flight. This exploration navigates through the intricacies of pre-flight briefings, unraveling the layers that contribute to a seamless, well-prepared, and ultimately safe flight experience.

1. The Foundation of Safety

Pre-flight briefings are not just a procedural formality; they are the bedrock of aviation safety. CFIs impress upon their students the gravity of this phase, emphasizing that meticulous attention to detail on the ground translates to confident and secure maneuvers in the air. Every checklist item, every piece of information conveyed during the pre-flight briefing serves as a protective shield against unforeseen challenges.

2. A Comprehensive Review of Flight Plans

The flight plan is the roadmap for the journey ahead. CFIs guide their students through a thorough examination of the flight plan during pre-flight briefings. Weather conditions, airspace considerations, alternate routes – each element is scrutinized to ensure that the plan is not just a route but a dynamic strategy that adapts to the ever-changing conditions of the sky.

3. Weather Wisdom: Interpreting the Skies

Weather, a fickle and potent force in aviation, demands careful interpretation. CFIs equip their students with the skills to decipher weather reports and forecasts. Pre-flight briefings become classrooms where the language of clouds, the significance of wind patterns, and the implications of atmospheric phenomena are unraveled. This weather wisdom is the armor that prepares pilots to navigate confidently through varying conditions.

4. Aircraft Systems: Knowing Your Bird

Pre-flight briefings extend beyond theoretical knowledge; they are hands-on sessions where students acquaint themselves with the intricacies of the aircraft. CFIs guide students through a systematic inspection of the aircraft systems – from engine checks to control surfaces. Understanding the mechanical heartbeat of the aircraft instills a sense of familiarity and confidence that resonates throughout the flight.

5. Emergency Preparedness: Expecting the Unexpected

The unforeseen is an inherent aspect of aviation. CFIs impress upon their students the importance of preparedness for emergencies. During pre-flight briefings, scenarios ranging from engine failures to unexpected weather changes are simulated and discussed. This mental preparedness ensures that when the unexpected does occur, pilots are not caught off guard but respond with poise and precision.

6. Crew Coordination and Communication

In the cockpit, communication is not just a luxury; it's a necessity. CFIs cultivate a culture of effective crew coordination during pre-flight briefings. From establishing clear communication protocols to practicing concise and accurate radio transmissions, these briefings set the tone for seamless collaboration between pilot and co-pilot.

7. Checklists: Rituals of Precision

Checklists are the rituals of precision in aviation. CFIs instill in their students the discipline of checklist adherence during pre-flight briefings. Each item, each step is not a mere task; it's a commitment to the systematic and thorough preparation that defines a successful flight.

8. Personal Readiness: Mind, Body, and Focus

The success of a flight extends beyond mechanical readiness to the mental and physical preparedness of the pilot. CFIs emphasize the importance of personal readiness during pre-flight briefings. From ensuring adequate rest to mental focus, these discussions contribute to a holistic approach to pilot well-being.

Post-Flight Debriefings: Learning from Every Experience

CERTAINLY, LET'S EXPLORE the crucial aspect of aviation with "Post-Flight Debriefings: Learning from Every Experience."

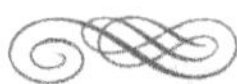

POST-FLIGHT DEBRIEFINGS: Learning from Every Experience

The hum of the engines fades, the aircraft touches down, and the sky surrenders to the runway below. Yet, for pilots, the journey doesn't conclude at landing; it extends into the realm of post-flight debriefings. An often-overlooked but indispensable facet of flight instruction, the post-flight debriefing is the cockpit's classroom after the wheels have kissed the tarmac. In these reflective sessions, Certified Flight Instructors (CFIs) guide their students through a process of analysis, critique, and continuous improvement.

1. The Art of Reflection

Post-flight debriefings transcend the realm of mere analysis; they are an art of reflection. CFIs encourage their students to revisit the flight mentally, dissecting each phase with a discerning eye. From takeoff to landing, every decision, every maneuver becomes a canvas for self-reflection.

2. Performance Assessment: Beyond the Numbers

Numbers on instruments tell one part of the story, but the true narrative lies in the nuanced assessment of performance. CFIs steer their students away from a mere numerical evaluation and delve into the qualitative aspects of the flight. Was the decision-making sound? Were maneuvers executed with precision? These are the questions that shape the post-flight discussion.

3. Weather and Airspace Challenges

The skies are unpredictable, and each flight presents its unique set of challenges. Post-flight debriefings serve as a platform to dissect how weather conditions and airspace complexities were navigated. CFIs guide their students through a retrospective journey, extracting lessons from the turbulence encountered or the strategic decisions made under changing weather patterns.

4. Scenario-Based Learning

Learning from real-life scenarios is a cornerstone of aviation education. CFIs employ post-flight debriefings to engage in scenario-based learning. "What if" becomes a powerful tool as students explore alternative decisions and responses, preparing them for the dynamic nature of future flights.

5. Communication Dynamics in the Cockpit

Effective communication is the heartbeat of flight safety. Post-flight debriefings extend beyond technicalities to explore the communication dynamics within the cockpit. CFIs facilitate discussions on how clear and concise communication contributed to a smooth flight or, conversely, how miscommunication may have introduced challenges.

6. Decision-Making under Pressure

The cockpit is a crucible where decisions are made under pressure. Post-flight debriefings provide a space for students to analyze their decision-making process. Whether it's navigating unexpected weather deviations or responding to in-flight anomalies, CFIs guide their students in dissecting the factors that influenced decisions and exploring alternatives for future improvement.

7. Continuous Improvement Mindset

Post-flight debriefings instill a mindset of continuous improvement. CFIs encourage their students not to view critiques as criticism but as catalysts for growth. Each debriefing becomes a stepping stone, propelling the pilot towards a higher standard of proficiency and a deeper understanding of aviation nuances.

8. Fatigue and Personal Well-being

A pilot's mental and physical well-being is as crucial post-flight as it is pre-flight. CFIs use debriefings to explore the impact of fatigue, stress, or external factors on performance. These discussions contribute to a holistic approach to pilot well-being, ensuring that future flights are undertaken with a clear and focused mind.

9. Goal Setting for Progress

Post-flight debriefings are not just about dissecting the past; they are also about charting the course for future progress. CFIs work with their students to set realistic yet challenging goals based on the insights gained. Whether refining specific maneuvers or enhancing decision-making skills, goal-setting becomes a compass for continuous advancement.

In the dynamic world of aviation, where each flight is a chapter in an ever-evolving narrative, post-flight debriefings stand as a testament to the commitment of CFIs and their students to unravel the lessons embedded in the skies.

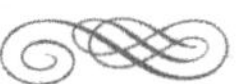

I hope you find this exploration of post-flight debriefings insightful and comprehensive. If you have any specific points you'd like to add or modify, feel free to let me know.

Incorporating Practical Tips for Effective Briefings

CERTAINLY, LET'S DELVE into the realm of effective briefings and how practical tips can enhance this critical aspect of flight instruction.

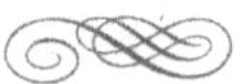

INCORPORATING PRACTICAL Tips for Effective Briefings

In the intricate dance of aviation instruction, where knowledge meets the cockpit, effective briefings emerge as a linchpin for success. The ability to convey information clearly, engage students, and set the stage for a safe and informed flight is an art that transcends the technicalities of the aircraft. Let's explore practical tips to elevate the art of briefings, creating an environment where understanding takes flight.

1. Clarity in Communication

At the core of every effective briefing is clarity in communication. Briefings are not a platform for jargon but an opportunity to translate complex concepts into digestible information. Instructors must distill intricate procedures into straightforward language, ensuring that students grasp the essentials without being overwhelmed by technicalities.

2. Engaging Visuals

The power of visuals in briefings cannot be overstated. Incorporating diagrams, charts, and interactive tools captures attention and enhances comprehension. Visual aids serve as a roadmap, guiding students through the intricacies of pre-flight checks, maneuvers, and emergency procedures with precision.

3. Interactive Discussions

Briefings should be dialogues, not monologues. Encourage interactive discussions that invite questions, scenarios, and active participation. This transforms briefings from passive information absorption sessions to dynamic exchanges where students feel empowered to seek clarification and delve deeper into concepts.

4. Real-World Scenarios

Bringing real-world scenarios into briefings adds a layer of practicality to theoretical knowledge. Instructors can draw from their experiences, illustrating how theoretical concepts manifest in actual flights. This connection to reality fosters a deeper understanding and better equips students for the dynamic challenges of aviation.

5. Tailoring to Individual Learning Styles

Every student absorbs information differently. Effective briefings acknowledge and cater to diverse learning styles. Whether visual, auditory, or kinesthetic, incorporating varied teaching methods ensures that every student receives information in a way that resonates with their preferred mode of learning.

6. Checklist Mastery

Checklists are the backbone of aviation procedures. Effective briefings should not only cover the items on a checklist but instill a mastery of its purpose and sequence. Instructors guide students through the logic behind each checklist item, fostering a comprehensive understanding that goes beyond rote memorization.

7. Dynamic Simulations

Incorporate dynamic simulations within briefings to simulate real-time decision-making. These simulations can range from emergency scenarios to in-flight adjustments. Practical tips within briefings might include step-by-step guides on handling unexpected situations, instilling confidence in students to navigate challenges effectively.

8. Utilize Technology

Embrace the technological tools available for modern briefings. From interactive apps to virtual reality simulations, leveraging technology enhances the briefing experience. This not only caters to the tech-savvy generation but also brings a dynamic and engaging element to the learning process.

9. Feedback Loop

Briefings are not just about imparting information; they are a continuous feedback loop. Instructors should actively seek feedback from students, gauging their comprehension and adjusting the briefing approach accordingly. This iterative process ensures that briefings evolve to meet the unique needs of each student.

10. Emphasis on Standard Operating Procedures (SOPs)

In the world of aviation, adherence to SOPs is paramount. Effective briefings emphasize the importance of following standard operating procedures rigorously. Instructors elucidate not just the "what" but the "why" behind each procedure, embedding a culture of safety and precision.

11. Time Management Strategies

Briefings are a delicate balance between thoroughness and efficiency. Instructors impart practical time management strategies, ensuring that briefings cover all essential elements without becoming overwhelming. This skill becomes invaluable as students progress to more complex flight scenarios.

12. Post-Briefing Review

The learning doesn't end with the briefing; it extends into the post-briefing review. Instructors guide students in reflecting on the briefing, reinforcing key concepts, and identifying areas that may require additional attention. This reflective practice cements knowledge and prepares students for practical application in the cockpit.

Effective briefings are not a mere prelude to flight; they are the cornerstone upon which a pilot's knowledge and confidence are built. By incorporating practical tips that transcend traditional instructional approaches, instructors can elevate briefings from routine information dissemination to transformative learning experiences.

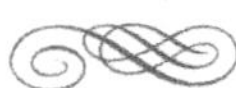

I TRUST THIS EXPLORATION provides a comprehensive guide to incorporating practical tips for effective briefings in aviation instruction. If there are specific areas you'd like to delve deeper into or any adjustments needed, feel free to let me know.

Chapter 7

Specialized Instruction and Endorsements

Tailoring Instruction for Different Aircraft Types

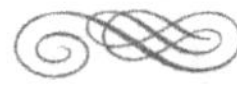

CERTAINLY, LET'S DELVE into the intricacies of tailoring instruction for different aircraft types, providing insights that cater to diverse aviation needs.

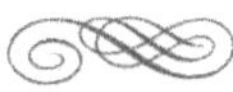

TAILORING INSTRUCTION for Different Aircraft Types

In the vast and dynamic world of aviation, the journey towards becoming a seasoned pilot involves mastering the nuances of various aircraft types. Each aircraft brings its own set of characteristics, quirks, and performance capabilities. As a flight instructor, the ability to tailor instruction to different aircraft types is not just a skill but a necessity. This guide aims to unravel the strategies and considerations involved in this tailored approach to instruction.

Understanding the Diversity of Aircraft

Before delving into instructional strategies, it's crucial to appreciate the diversity that exists among aircraft. From light trainers to complex jets, each category demands a unique set of skills and knowledge. Understanding the aerodynamic principles, systems, and operational intricacies specific to different aircraft types lays the foundation for effective instruction.

Adapting to Training Needs

Tailoring instruction begins with recognizing the training needs inherent to each aircraft category. For novice pilots stepping into the cockpit of a small trainer, the focus might be on fundamental maneuvers, basic navigation, and understanding aircraft systems. On the other hand, transitioning to larger, more complex aircraft demands a deeper grasp of advanced avionics, high-altitude considerations, and intricate systems management.

Customizing Lesson Plans

Lesson plans act as the roadmap for aviation instruction. Tailoring these plans involves customizing content to suit the characteristics of the aircraft in focus. Lessons for a single-engine propeller plane might emphasize fundamental maneuvers like stalls and steep turns, while lessons for a multi-engine jet could delve into complex systems, crew coordination, and high-altitude procedures.

Simulator Integration

Simulators play a pivotal role in tailoring instruction for different aircraft types. They provide a controlled environment where pilots can familiarize themselves with the specific handling and systems of diverse aircraft. Flight instructors leverage simulator sessions to bridge the gap between theory and practical application, ensuring that pilots are well-prepared for the unique challenges each aircraft presents.

Emphasizing Safety Procedures

Safety is a non-negotiable aspect of aviation, and tailoring instruction involves a meticulous focus on safety procedures relevant to the aircraft at hand. Whether it's emergency procedures, abnormal situations, or specific checklist protocols, instructors guide pilots through the intricacies of responding to challenges in a manner aligned with the characteristics of the aircraft type.

Navigational Variances

Different aircraft types often come with variations in navigational equipment and procedures. Instructors tailor navigation lessons to encompass the specific avionics and navigation systems utilized by the aircraft. This includes understanding GPS systems, VOR navigation, and instrument approach procedures that align with the capabilities of the aircraft being flown.

Crew Resource Management (CRM)

For pilots transitioning to larger aircraft requiring crew coordination, CRM becomes a crucial aspect of instruction. Emphasizing effective communication, workload management, and situational awareness tailored to the multi-crew environment ensures a seamless integration into the dynamics of larger, more complex aircraft.

Practical Application in Cross-Country Flights

Tailored instruction extends beyond the basics to practical application. Cross-country flights present an opportunity to expose pilots to the unique considerations of navigating diverse landscapes, airports, and airspace. Instructors guide pilots in planning and executing cross-country flights, considering factors such as fuel planning, weather variations, and diverse airport facilities.

Continuous Assessment and Feedback

Tailoring instruction involves a continuous feedback loop. Flight instructors conduct regular assessments that gauge a pilot's proficiency in handling the specific aircraft type. Constructive feedback guides pilots in refining their skills, addressing weaknesses, and building confidence in their ability to navigate the complexities of the chosen aircraft.

Transition Training Programs

For pilots transitioning between aircraft types, structured transition training programs become invaluable. These programs, tailored to address the specific challenges of moving from one category of aircraft to another, provide a systematic approach to building competence and confidence in the new environment.

Leveraging Technology

In the modern era of aviation, technology offers tools that aid in tailoring instruction. Flight instructors integrate advanced avionics training software, virtual reality simulations, and interactive learning platforms to enhance the educational experience. These technologies provide a dynamic and engaging approach to understanding the intricacies of different aircraft types.

Conclusion

Tailoring instruction for different aircraft types is an intricate dance that requires a deep understanding of aviation's diverse landscape. Flight instructors, serving as mentors and guides, play a pivotal role in shaping the next generation of aviators. By recognizing the unique demands of each aircraft type, customizing lesson plans, and embracing evolving technologies, instructors empower pilots to navigate the skies with skill, precision, and a profound appreciation for the complexities of flight.

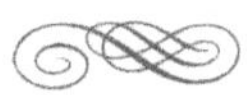

I TRUST THIS EXPLORATION provides a comprehensive guide to tailoring instruction for different aircraft types. If you have specific areas you'd like to delve deeper into or any adjustments needed, feel free to let me know.

Understanding and Issuing Endorsements

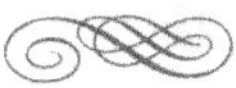

CERTAINLY, LET'S DELVE into the intricate world of understanding and issuing endorsements in aviation, providing insights and guidance that resonate with both novice pilots and seasoned professionals.

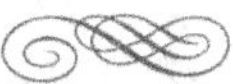

UNDERSTANDING AND ISSUING Endorsements in Aviation

Aviation, with its vast array of regulations and requirements, demands a nuanced understanding of endorsements—those crucial stamps of approval that signify a pilot's competence in specific areas. Whether you're an aspiring aviator or an experienced flight instructor, comprehending the intricacies of endorsements is paramount to navigating the skies safely and efficiently.

The Significance of Endorsements

Endorsements in aviation serve as a testament to a pilot's proficiency in various skills, maneuvers, or aircraft. They are not just bureaucratic formalities; rather, they are tangible validations of a pilot's ability to handle specific challenges and scenarios. From complex maneuvers to transitioning between aircraft types, endorsements are the badges of expertise that adorn a pilot's record.

Basic Endorsements for Student Pilots

For those embarking on the exhilarating journey of flight, the initial phase often involves student pilot endorsements. These endorsements cover the foundational skills required for safe solo flight. Whether it's the first solo flight endorsement or specific endorsements for cross-country flights or night operations, each signifies a milestone in a student pilot's progression.

High-Performance and Complex Aircraft Endorsements

As pilots advance in their training, endorsements extend to encompass high-performance and complex aircraft. Understanding the intricacies of these endorsements is vital for those aiming to explore the capabilities of more powerful and sophisticated flying machines. High-performance endorsements typically involve aircraft with engines exceeding 200 horsepower, while complex endorsements are specific to aircraft with retractable landing gear, flaps, and a controllable-pitch propeller.

Tailwheel and Seaplane Endorsements

The diversity of aviation is reflected in specialized endorsements for tailwheel and seaplane operations. Tailwheel aircraft, with their unique handling characteristics during takeoff and landing, necessitate specific training and endorsements. Similarly, the allure of water-based operations draws pilots to pursue seaplane endorsements, adding versatility to their flying repertoire.

Instrument and Multi-Engine Endorsements

Delving into more advanced realms, instrument and multi-engine endorsements open doors to new horizons. The instrument rating endorsement signifies a pilot's ability to navigate and operate an aircraft solely by reference to instruments—a critical skill for flying in varied weather conditions. Multi-engine endorsements, on the other hand, mark a transition to aircraft with multiple engines, demanding heightened coordination and systems management.

Flight Instructor Endorsements

For those aspiring to guide the next generation of aviators, flight instructor endorsements become paramount. These encompass not only the endorsement to instruct but also additional endorsements for specific instructional privileges. From teaching instrument flying to providing complex aircraft instruction, flight instructors play a pivotal role in shaping the skills and knowledge of aspiring pilots.

Navigating Endorsements for Recurrent Training

Aviation is a dynamic field, and staying current is imperative. Endorsements for recurrent training, such as those related to instrument proficiency checks (IPCs), ensure that pilots maintain the skills necessary for safe and proficient flight. These endorsements underscore the commitment to ongoing education and proficiency.

The Role of Flight Instructors in Issuing Endorsements

Flight instructors wield a profound responsibility in the endorsement process. Beyond being educators, they are evaluators who assess a pilot's readiness for specific endorsements. Precision, attention to detail, and a thorough understanding of regulatory requirements define the role of a flight instructor in endorsing a pilot's logbook.

Challenges and Considerations in Issuing Endorsements

While endorsements are a mark of accomplishment, they come with challenges. Flight instructors must navigate the delicate balance of ensuring pilots meet regulatory standards while fostering a positive and constructive learning environment. Tailoring instruction to address specific areas of improvement is key to issuing endorsements that truly reflect a pilot's preparedness.

Evolving Technologies and Endorsements

In the era of advanced avionics and technology, the landscape of endorsements is evolving. Pilots are increasingly required to demonstrate proficiency in utilizing modern navigation systems and electronic flight bags. Flight instructors must adapt their training methods to encompass these technological advancements, ensuring pilots are equipped to operate in contemporary aviation environments.

Conclusion

Understanding and issuing endorsements in aviation is a dynamic process that mirrors the diverse facets of flying. Whether you're a student pilot embarking on your first solo flight or an experienced aviator pursuing advanced endorsements, each step represents a milestone in your aviation journey. Flight instructors, as mentors and evaluators, play an instrumental role in guiding pilots through this intricate web of endorsements, ensuring that each stamp in the logbook is a testament to competence, proficiency, and a passion for safe and skillful flight.

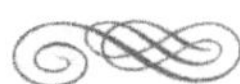

I TRUST THIS EXPLORATION provides a comprehensive guide to understanding and issuing endorsements in aviation. Should you have specific areas you'd like to delve deeper into or any adjustments needed, feel free to let me know.

Navigating the World of Type Ratings and Additional Certifications

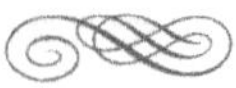

CERTAINLY, LET'S EMBARK on a journey through the intricate landscape of type ratings and additional certifications in the aviation realm, unraveling the complexities and significance that these qualifications hold for pilots worldwide.

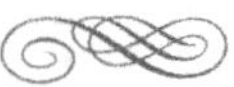

NAVIGATING THE WORLD of Type Ratings and Additional Certifications

Aviation, with its ever-evolving technology and diverse aircraft, demands pilots to navigate a maze of qualifications, with type ratings and additional certifications standing as pivotal waypoints on the journey to mastery. In this exploration, we delve into the intricacies of these certifications, understanding their importance, the avenues they open, and the commitment they signify.

1. Type Ratings: Unveiling the Aircraft-Specific Expertise

Type ratings are the hallmark of a pilot's proficiency in operating specific aircraft models. Unlike a generic pilot's license, a type rating is aircraft-specific, reflecting a pilot's in-depth understanding of the systems, procedures, and nuances unique to a particular aircraft. Whether it's a jumbo jet, a sleek corporate aircraft, or a cutting-edge airliner, obtaining a type rating is akin to unlocking the doors to an exclusive club, signifying a pilot's capability to command sophisticated flying machines.

2. The Training Odyssey: From General to Specific

The journey towards a type rating is a structured odyssey. Pilots typically commence their training with a private pilot's license, gradually advancing through commercial and instrument ratings. While these provide a foundation, type ratings elevate the training to a granular level. Ground school education, simulator sessions, and actual flight hours in the specific aircraft are integral components, ensuring that pilots emerge not only with the technical knowledge but also the practical skills required to handle the aircraft competently.

3. The Realm of Multi-Engine Aircraft

Multi-engine aircraft present a distinct realm within aviation. Pilots seeking to operate these aircraft acquire multi-engine ratings, signifying their ability to manage the complexities of multiple engines, systems, and the associated challenges. This certification is foundational for those aspiring to fly larger, more powerful aircraft that require a heightened level of skill and coordination.

4. Additional Certifications: Expanding Horizons

Beyond type ratings, pilots often pursue additional certifications that broaden their capabilities and open doors to specialized aviation domains. Some of these certifications include:

- Instrument Rating: Proficiency in flying solely by reference to instruments, crucial for navigating through adverse weather conditions.

- Flight Instructor Certificate: For those with a passion for teaching, this certification allows pilots to guide and mentor aspiring aviators, contributing to the growth of the aviation community.

- Airline Transport Pilot (ATP) Certificate: The pinnacle of pilot certifications, the ATP signifies the highest level of qualification, essential for commanding commercial airliners.

- Seaplane Rating: Adding a splash of versatility, this certification allows pilots to operate aircraft on water, expanding their repertoire of flying environments.

5. The Regulatory Tapestry: Navigating Federal Aviation Administration (FAA) Requirements

In the United States, the Federal Aviation Administration (FAA) plays a central role in defining the requirements for type ratings and additional certifications. Navigating this regulatory tapestry demands meticulous attention to detail and adherence to stringent standards. Pilots must meet not only the flight hour prerequisites but also demonstrate a profound understanding of aeronautical knowledge through rigorous examinations.

6. Currency, Renewals, and Ongoing Training

Earning a type rating or additional certification is not a static achievement but a commitment to continuous learning. Pilots must maintain currency, staying abreast of evolving technologies, procedures, and regulations. Renewals and recurrent training sessions ensure that pilots remain at the forefront of safety and proficiency, reflecting the industry's dedication to a culture of excellence.

7. The Global Perspective: International Standards and Harmonization

In an era of global connectivity, aviation certifications often transcend national borders. International agreements and harmonization efforts strive to standardize aviation qualifications, facilitating the seamless movement of pilots across diverse airspace. These agreements, such as those established by the International Civil Aviation Organization (ICAO), underscore the collaborative nature of the aviation industry in ensuring universal safety and competency standards.

8. The Pilot's Odyssey: From Aspiration to Mastery

Embarking on the journey of type ratings and additional certifications is akin to an odyssey for pilots—one that evolves from the aspiration of taking flight to the mastery of commanding advanced aircraft. Each certification attained is not merely a badge on a pilot's uniform but a testament to their dedication, perseverance, and passion for the skies.

Conclusion

In navigating the world of type ratings and additional certifications, pilots traverse a path marked by precision, expertise, and an unwavering commitment to safety. From type-specific endorsements to broader certifications that encompass diverse facets of aviation, the journey reflects the profound evolution of a pilot's skills and knowledge. As we soar through this exploration, it becomes evident that the world above is not just a vast expanse of airspace but a canvas where pilots paint their stories of achievement, one certification at a time.

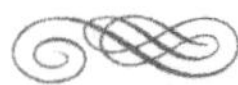

I TRUST THIS EXTENSIVE exploration provides a comprehensive guide to the world of type ratings and additional certifications in aviation. If there are specific areas you'd like to delve deeper into or any adjustments needed, feel free to let me know.

Chapter 8

Maintaining Professionalism

Professionalism in and out of the Cockpit

Certainly, let's explore the nuanced realm of professionalism within and beyond the cockpit, unraveling the intricacies that define the conduct of aviators both in the skies and on solid ground.

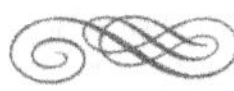

PROFESSIONALISM IN and out of the Cockpit

Aviation, often revered as the epitome of precision and discipline, extends beyond the mere mechanics of flight. It is an embodiment of professionalism that permeates every facet of a pilot's journey—whether navigating the complex controls of an aircraft or interacting with colleagues, passengers, and the aviation community at large.

1. The Essence of Cockpit Professionalism

Precision in Execution:

At the heart of cockpit professionalism lies an unwavering commitment to precision. Aviators, akin to conductors orchestrating a symphony, navigate the skies with meticulous attention to detail. From pre-flight checklists to executing intricate maneuvers, the cockpit is a domain where every action is deliberate, calculated, and carried out with the utmost precision.

Crisis Management:

Professionalism in the cockpit is perhaps most profoundly tested during moments of crisis. Whether faced with adverse weather conditions, technical malfunctions, or unforeseen challenges, aviators must embody calm and composed decision-making. The ability to manage crises without compromising safety is a hallmark of professionalism that extends far beyond technical expertise.

Effective Communication:

In the cockpit, communication is not merely a tool; it is a lifeline. Professional aviators master the art of concise, clear, and unambiguous communication. The cockpit crew operates as a tightly-knit team, and effective communication is imperative for the safe and efficient execution of flight operations.

2. Extending Professionalism Beyond the Skies

Interpersonal Skills:

Beyond the confines of the cockpit, aviators are ambassadors of the skies. Professionalism extends to interpersonal skills, emphasizing respect, courtesy, and empathy. From interactions with ground crew to engaging with passengers, aviators represent not just a profession but a culture of excellence.

Continuous Learning and Adaptability:

True professionals recognize that learning is a lifelong journey. The aviation landscape is dynamic, with advancements in technology, regulatory changes, and evolving best practices. Aviators exhibit professionalism by embracing continuous learning, staying abreast of industry developments, and adapting to new challenges.

Ethical Decision-Making:

The aviation community places a premium on ethical conduct. Aviators are entrusted with the safety of those on board, and professionalism demands ethical decision-making, even in the face of external pressures. Upholding the highest standards of integrity is not just a requirement; it is an intrinsic part of being a professional aviator.

3. Navigating Cultural Sensitivities

Global Perspectives:

In an era of global connectivity, aviators often traverse diverse cultural landscapes. Professionalism encompasses an understanding of cultural nuances, fostering an environment of inclusivity and respect. Aviators navigate not only through airspace but also through a rich tapestry of global cultures.

Language Proficiency:

Effective communication transcends linguistic barriers. Professional aviators often operate in environments where multiple languages are spoken. Proficiency in English, recognized as the international language of aviation, is a cornerstone of professionalism, ensuring a common platform for communication.

4. The Regulatory Framework of Professionalism

Regulatory Compliance:

Professionalism within aviation is not a vague ideal; it is codified within a robust regulatory framework. Aviation authorities, such as the Federal Aviation Administration (FAA) in the United States, define standards of professionalism that encompass everything from licensing requirements to adherence to operational procedures. Aviators navigate their careers within this regulatory framework, reinforcing the importance of professionalism.

Safety as a Professional Imperative:

Above all, professionalism in aviation is inseparable from the commitment to safety. Aviators recognize that safety is not a standalone objective but an integral part of being a professional. Safety protocols, adherence to regulations, and a proactive approach to risk management are emblematic of the professionalism that underpins every flight.

5. Personal Wellness: The Human Dimension of Professionalism

Physical and Mental Well-being:

Professionalism demands more than technical prowess; it encompasses the holistic well-being of aviators. Physical and mental fitness are integral components. Pilots prioritize health, recognizing that their personal wellness directly impacts their ability to execute their professional duties with precision and resilience.

Work-Life Balance:

The aviation industry, known for its demanding schedules, underscores the importance of work-life balance. Professionals recognize that maintaining a healthy equilibrium between professional responsibilities and personal life is not just beneficial but essential for sustained excellence.

6. Towards a Sustainable Future: Environmental Stewardship

Environmental Responsibility:

As custodians of the skies, aviators embrace environmental stewardship as a facet of professionalism. Adherence to fuel-efficient practices, exploring sustainable aviation fuels, and minimizing the ecological footprint are manifestations of a commitment to a sustainable and responsible aviation industry.

Conclusion

In traversing the realms of professionalism within and beyond the cockpit, aviators embark on a journey that transcends the technicalities of flight. It is a commitment to precision, ethical conduct, and the well-being of both individuals and the global community. Professionalism is not a static destination but a continuous evolution—an unwavering dedication to excellence that defines the very essence of aviation.

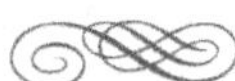

I HOPE THIS EXPLORATION into professionalism within and beyond the cockpit provides the depth and detail you were seeking. If you have any specific areas you'd like to delve into further or if there are adjustments needed, feel free to let me know.

Continuous Learning: Staying Updated with Industry Changes

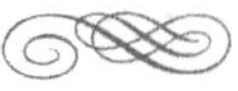

CERTAINLY, LET'S EXPLORE the significance of continuous learning in the dynamic realm of aviation, focusing on the imperative of staying updated with industry changes.

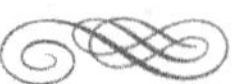

CONTINUOUS LEARNING: Navigating the Ever-Evolving Skies

In the vast expanse of aviation, where technology, regulations, and best practices are in a constant state of flux, the commitment to continuous learning stands as an unwavering beacon for aviators. This journey into the skies is not a static one—it's a perpetual odyssey of adaptation, where staying updated with industry changes is not just a choice but a professional imperative.

1. The Dynamic Landscape of Aviation

Technological Advancements:

The aviation industry is a hotbed of technological innovation. From advancements in avionics and navigation systems to the integration of artificial intelligence, staying abreast of the latest technological developments is crucial. Continuous learning allows aviators to harness the power of cutting-edge technology, enhancing the safety and efficiency of flight operations.

Regulatory Shifts:

Regulations within the aviation sector are subject to evolution. Whether it's updates in safety protocols, changes in airspace regulations, or modifications to licensing requirements, aviators must stay attuned to regulatory shifts. Continuous learning ensures compliance with the latest standards, fostering a culture of safety and adherence to legal frameworks.

Global Perspectives:

Aviation is a global enterprise, and the ability to navigate diverse international landscapes is contingent upon an understanding of global aviation trends. Continuous learning provides aviators with insights into international best practices, emerging trends, and the cultural nuances that define the global aviation community.

2. Professional Development: A Lifelong Journey

Type Ratings and Specializations:

Aviation professionals often seek to expand their repertoire of skills through type ratings and specializations. Whether acquiring expertise in flying specific aircraft types or delving into specialized areas such as aerobatics or cargo operations, continuous learning opens avenues for professional growth and diversification.

Safety Management Systems (SMS):

In an era where safety is paramount, the integration of Safety Management Systems (SMS) is a pivotal advancement. Aviators engage in continuous learning to understand and implement SMS effectively. This proactive approach to risk management enhances safety culture within aviation organizations.

Human Factors and Crew Resource Management (CRM):

Understanding human factors and mastering Crew Resource Management (CRM) are integral components of continuous learning. Aviators delve into psychological aspects, communication strategies, and teamwork dynamics to ensure the human element is optimized for safe and efficient flight operations.

3. Adapting to Environmental Imperatives

Sustainable Aviation Practices:

The aviation industry is increasingly embracing sustainability. Aviators engage in continuous learning to adopt eco-friendly practices, including fuel-efficient flying techniques, exploring alternative fuels, and contributing to the broader goal of mitigating the environmental impact of aviation.

Climate and Weather Trends:

Climate change introduces new dynamics to weather patterns, affecting flight operations. Continuous learning in meteorology and climate science enables aviators to anticipate and navigate through changing weather conditions, ensuring the safety and comfort of passengers.

4. The Role of Simulators and Virtual Learning

Simulators for Realistic Training:

Simulators have become invaluable tools for continuous learning. Aviators immerse themselves in realistic scenarios, honing their skills and decision-making abilities in a controlled environment. Simulators offer a safe space to practice emergency procedures, refine flying techniques, and enhance overall proficiency.

Virtual Learning Platforms:

With the advent of digital technology, virtual learning platforms have become instrumental in continuous education. Aviators access online courses, webinars, and e-learning modules to stay updated on industry trends, regulations, and specialized topics. These platforms facilitate learning at one's own pace, fostering a culture of self-directed continuous improvement.

5. Building a Learning Organization

Organizational Culture:

Continuous learning is not confined to individual aviators; it permeates the organizational culture. Aviation entities committed to excellence prioritize ongoing education for their staff. This commitment ensures that the collective knowledge base of the organization evolves, creating a resilient and adaptive entity capable of meeting the challenges of the dynamic aviation landscape.

Knowledge Sharing:

Aviation thrives on the synergy of shared knowledge. Continuous learning extends beyond individual pursuits to collaborative efforts within the aviation community. Aviators participate in forums, conferences, and knowledge-sharing platforms, contributing to a collective reservoir of expertise that benefits the entire industry.

Conclusion

In the ever-evolving skies, continuous learning is not just a practice; it's a mindset—an unwavering commitment to excellence and safety. Aviators who embrace continuous learning are not merely passengers on the journey of aviation; they are the navigators, charting a course through the complexities of an industry in perpetual motion.

Navigating Challenges and Ethical Considerations

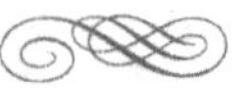

CERTAINLY, LET'S DELVE into the intricate landscape of navigating challenges and ethical considerations in a professional context.

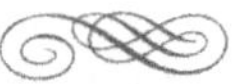

NAVIGATING CHALLENGES and Ethical Considerations: A Professional Odyssey

In the realm of any profession, the journey is seldom a straight and unobstructed path. Challenges, both expected and unforeseen, pepper the professional landscape, requiring individuals to navigate them with a deft touch and a keen ethical compass. This exploration will not only identify common challenges faced across various professions but also dissect the ethical considerations that act as guiding stars in overcoming these obstacles.

1. Identifying Common Professional Challenges

a. Technological Advancements:

As technology continues its relentless march forward, professionals often find themselves grappling with the need to adapt swiftly. Whether it's mastering new software, understanding automation, or incorporating artificial intelligence into workflows, staying technologically relevant is a constant challenge.

b. Workplace Dynamics:

Navigating the complex terrain of workplace relationships and dynamics presents another set of challenges. Balancing collaboration with individual contribution, managing conflicts, and fostering a healthy work environment demand a nuanced approach from professionals across sectors.

c. Regulatory Complexity:

Many professions operate within a web of regulations and compliance standards. Staying abreast of these evolving rules while ensuring that daily operations align with legal requirements poses an ongoing challenge. Failure to navigate this successfully can have legal and ethical implications.

d. Time Management and Work-Life Balance:

In a fast-paced world, time becomes a precious commodity. Professionals often face the challenge of balancing demanding work schedules with personal and family commitments. Maintaining a healthy work-life balance is not only a personal challenge but also an organizational imperative for sustainable productivity.

e. Globalization and Cultural Sensitivity:

In an interconnected world, professionals frequently find themselves working in diverse and global environments. Bridging cultural gaps, understanding international business etiquette, and fostering cultural sensitivity are challenges faced by those navigating the globalized landscape.

2. The Ethical Imperative: A Guiding Light

a. Ethical Decision-Making:

When confronted with challenges, the decisions professionals make often extend beyond immediate problem-solving; they shape the ethical fabric of the organization. Ethical decision-making involves considering the impact on stakeholders, maintaining transparency, and upholding principles of integrity and fairness.

b. Balancing Competing Interests:

Ethical challenges sometimes arise from competing interests within an organization. Professionals must navigate these conflicts by ensuring decisions align with the organization's values and serve the greater good, even when faced with conflicting priorities.

c. Honesty and Transparency:

Facing challenges head-on requires a commitment to honesty and transparency. Professionals must communicate openly about issues, risks, and potential setbacks. This not only builds trust within the organization but also fosters a culture of accountability.

d. Respecting Diversity and Inclusion:

Cultural sensitivity and inclusivity are integral components of ethical behavior. Professionals must actively work to understand and respect diverse perspectives, fostering an inclusive environment that values the contributions of individuals from various backgrounds.

e. Responsibility to Society:

Beyond the immediate organizational context, professionals bear a broader responsibility to society. This involves considering the environmental impact of business practices, contributing positively to communities, and upholding ethical standards that transcend organizational boundaries.

3. Case Studies: Real-World Challenges and Ethical Responses

a. Data Privacy in the Digital Age:

As organizations collect vast amounts of data, professionals face the challenge of ensuring data privacy. Ethical responses involve implementing robust cybersecurity measures, obtaining informed consent, and aligning practices with data protection laws.

b. Workplace Harassment:

Navigating challenges related to workplace harassment demands an ethical commitment to creating a safe and respectful environment. This involves implementing stringent anti-harassment policies, providing clear reporting mechanisms, and fostering a culture that condemns such behaviors.

c. Environmental Sustainability:

Professionals involved in industries impacting the environment face the challenge of balancing business interests with ecological responsibility. Ethical responses may include adopting sustainable practices, investing in green technologies, and actively participating in environmental conservation initiatives.

4. Cultivating Ethical Leadership

a. Leading by Example:

Ethical challenges often require leadership to set the tone. Leaders who exemplify ethical behavior create a culture where professionals feel empowered to navigate challenges transparently and ethically.

b. Providing Ethical Guidance:

Organizations benefit from establishing clear ethical guidelines and providing resources for professionals to seek guidance. Ethical considerations should be integrated into training programs, emphasizing the importance of principled decision-making.

5. Conclusion: A Journey of Integrity

In the vast and intricate landscape of professional challenges, navigating with integrity remains the compass that ensures individuals and organizations stay true to their purpose. Ethical considerations, far from being mere guidelines, become the very essence of professional identity—a commitment to doing what is right, even in the face of adversity.

Conclusion

Conclusion: Navigating the Professional Landscape with Expertise and Integrity

In concluding our exploration of the multifaceted realm of professional development, the intricate tapestry of challenges, ethical considerations, and the pursuit of excellence becomes apparent. As we traverse the vast expanse of industries and professions, certain overarching principles emerge—principles that underscore the significance of continuous learning, ethical leadership, and adaptability in the face of ever-evolving landscapes.

1. Embracing Continuous Learning: The Lifelong Journey

The journey of a professional is, fundamentally, a journey of continuous learning. In an era where technological advancements reshape industries at an unprecedented pace, the commitment to staying updated is not merely a choice but a necessity. Professionals must embrace a mindset of perpetual curiosity, seeking out opportunities for upskilling and reskilling to remain relevant and effective contributors to their fields.

2. The Ethical Compass: Guiding the Professional Odyssey

Ethics stands as the unwavering compass that steers professionals through the challenges and dilemmas inherent in their journeys. Navigating with integrity involves making decisions that reflect a commitment to honesty, transparency, and responsibility to society. As we've explored various challenges—whether they be related to technology, workplace dynamics, or environmental sustainability—the ethical imperative emerges as the bedrock upon which resilient and principled professional conduct is built.

3. Diversity and Inclusion: Catalysts for Innovation

Recognizing the value of diversity and inclusion is not merely a contemporary buzz phrase but a core principle that propels organizations toward innovation and excellence. Professionals must actively cultivate environments that celebrate differences, fostering a culture where everyone feels heard, valued, and empowered to contribute their unique perspectives.

4. Leadership: Forging the Path Ahead

Leadership, in its truest form, is not just about directing others; it's about inspiring them to navigate challenges with resilience and ethical acuity. Ethical leaders set the tone for organizational culture, providing the guidance and resources needed for professionals to excel and contribute meaningfully.

5. Adapting to Change: The Essence of Resilience

Change is an ever-present companion on the professional journey. Whether it's adapting to new technologies, navigating shifts in workplace dynamics, or responding to global challenges, professionals must embody resilience. The ability to not only weather change but to harness it as a catalyst for growth and improvement becomes a hallmark of successful professionals.

6. A Call to Action: Crafting a Future of Excellence

As we conclude this exploration, it's not merely an endpoint but a call to action—a call for professionals to forge a future of excellence. It's a commitment to embodying the principles of continuous learning, ethical conduct, inclusivity, and resilience. The professional landscape is ever-evolving, and those who embrace these principles not only navigate challenges effectively but also contribute to shaping a future where expertise meets integrity.

In essence, the professional journey is not a solitary endeavor but a collective odyssey where individuals, guided by expertise and integrity, contribute to a broader narrative of progress and excellence. Through our shared commitment to knowledge, ethical conduct, and adaptability, we propel ourselves and our professions toward horizons yet unexplored.

As you reflect on the insights shared in this comprehensive exploration, may they serve as beacons lighting your path through the intricate and dynamic world of professional development. Your journey, shaped by expertise and integrity, unfolds as a narrative of impact, resilience, and lasting significance.

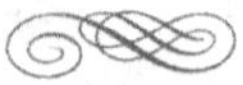

I TRUST THIS CONCLUSION encapsulates the essence of our exploration. If there are specific elements you'd like to emphasize or any adjustments needed, feel free to let me know.